"From a small seed
a mighty trunk
may grow."

-Aeschylus

INTRODUCTION

I've known for a long time I was passionate about understanding the mind and how it works. When I began pursuing my undergraduate degree in Journalism, I did it based on my skills, but I knew deep down that I was supposed to help build solutions for people to overcome trauma. I didn't know exactly how to do that, but I was ready for just about any adventure that was to come. Or, so I thought.

While in my junior year of college, I began to have panic attacks. I felt strange sensations in my arms and legs, like pins and needles. I had no grid for what was happening to my body: shallow breathing, racing thoughts, cold sweats, and limpness all over. They didn't stop that morning. In fact, they began to increase in intensity and frequency.

Shortly after I graduated college, I began to have feelings of depression as I learned my "new normal". I was running my own company, undergoing major life transition moving abroad and then back to Dallas, and figuring out what to do with my life. I didn't know that my gut, which had begun acting up a year or so prior, was directly involved in perpetuating the emotions that themselves needed support and balancing.

As I attempted to sort out my life, my feelings didn't seem to improve. One day, I arrived at my parents' home and my mom handed me a couple of bottles of essential oils she had just been introduced to: peppermint and lavender. My eyes rolled and I believe I told her aloud cynically that this would last "about six months before the fad wears off and you abandon yet another product." To me, it was like anything else she had brought home and used for a brief time before forgetting about it.

I didn't pay the bottles of oil much thought at all until a few months later when my older sister, who is typically the greater cynic than I, began chasing people around the house asking if they had certain ailments before rubbing peppermint essential oil on them. It was then I realized there was something there. Typically, I was the one who was the "early adopter" so if my sister could get on board, surely there was something to these essential oils! I needed to get on really fast or I'd miss out. I tried two bottles of oil, a blend for balancing emotions and a blend for digestion. The emotional blend I used one time in the middle of a panic attack and it stopped immediately! Needless to say, I was convinced.

My collection of essential oils grew steadily as I experimented with different things. I began noticing changes in my body and emotions and soon the panic attacks stopped altogether. During this same time, I made some slight dietary changes and also began seeing a counselor and pursuing the inner healing I desperately needed. I believe it is because of my multi-pronged approach that I received the healing. I can't point to any particular thing that was a silver bullet. Each tool in my healing toolbox was beneficial in restoring my spirit, soul, and body to wholeness. It's because of my own path that I have a value and appreciation for everyone's unique healing journey.

After experiencing essential oils, I knew first-hand that they worked powerfully, but I wasn't satisfied with the cliché answers as to why. So, I began to do more research. I read, attended classes, listened to countless experienced individuals, and kept experimenting on my own.

Not long after discovering essential oils, I began my graduate studies at the University of Texas at Dallas in Applied Cognition and Neuroscience. I loved every single moment of my grad school experience. I loved that I could learn not just the psychological theories of the mind, but I could be in the thick of discovering the "how and why" behind the structure and function of the brain. It didn't take me long after entering graduate school to begin asking questions to my professors and the researchers around me. I'd ask them about their experience with essential oils, what they were finding in the research, and how essential oils might be able to benefit and be developed for treatments for the mind and the brain. It also didn't take me very long after asking to realize that they had no idea what I was talking about. Most of them either dismissed it as "snake oil" or they wanted to see the quantitative research. Very few had any experience with essential oils at all. I began to see a clear disconnect between the essential oil and naturally-minded community that was having amazing breakthroughs, and the medical community full of researchers, doctors, and brilliant scientists who were also finding solutions for people, but were still missing keys which could revolutionize how they treated patients. I was in the midst of both communities and I loved them equally. So, I made it my mission to do my own research and help bridge the gap between the natural health community and the allopathic (Western) model of medicine. That's where this book was born.

Mind Your Brain Lite is designed to bring quantifiable data from the research community together with crystallized knowledge in an accessible form to explain how and why essential oils work to affect the structure and function of the brain and mind as well as give a framework for the process of inner healing. So, welcome! And thanks for minding your brain!

xo, *Elizabeth Erickson*

ECOSYSTEMS

Just like a plant lives in a highly dynamic environment, humans also live in an ecosystem. We are adaptable, resilient, and much stronger than we know.

Like plants, many things affect us including positive input (i.e. nutrients, healthy relationships, and natural resources). Negative things can also affect us including stress, trauma, broken relationships, lack of nurture and care. Each variable affects the makeup of who we are. The greater the negative input, the greater the negative expression. The more positive the input, the more positive the expression. The same is true as we approach talking about the mind and the brain.

If we just try to fix one variable or apply an essential oil or particular therapy method without examining the entire ecosystem of our brains and bodies, it's likely we won't get the full benefit available to us if we fail to look at our lives holistically.

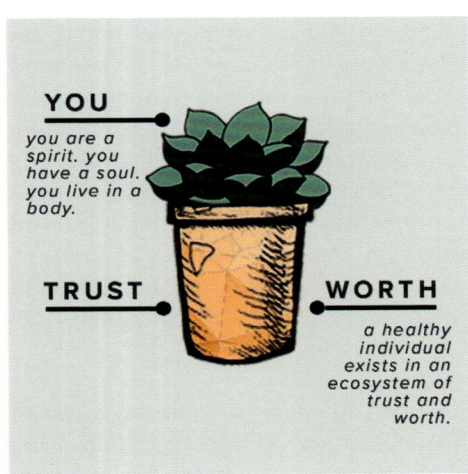

YOU

you are a spirit. you have a soul. you live in a body.

TRUST   WORTH

a healthy individual exists in an ecosystem of trust and worth.

As we approach healing the brain and the mind, it's important to note we are working from a theoretical model named "Pneuma, Psyche, Soma", the Greek words for spirit, soul, and body.

You are a spirit, you have a soul, and you live in a body and are designed to flow in that order.

In order to have a vibrant life, the "soil" of your spirit, soul, and body must contain two key elements: trust and worth. You can have one without the other, but you won't have vibrancy if you don't combine both.

THE BASICS OF ESSENTIAL OILS

Essential oils should not be approached just like a medicine. They are highly complex molecular compounds that are dynamic and work in dynamic environments. Essential oils are extracted from raw plant material either by a specialized distillation process of the plant matter or for some plants (ike citrus fruits) by cold pressing from the rind. They are volatile, water-insoluble oily liquids that are usually colorless and are different than lipid oils in both their molecular structure and volatility.

Essential oils serve plants and humans in 4 main ways:
1. They bring nourishment and participate in metabolic processes
2. They help reduce inflammation and combat infection
3. They help provide and balance hormones (ligands)
4. They help repair damage at the cellular level

In general, there are three main ways to use essential oils:
1. Aromatically through direct inhalation or passive diffusion

Direct inhalation usually means applying an oil to your hand, holding over the nose, and inhaling.

Passive diffusion can happen in a variety of ways, including a special diffuser, clothing, or jewelry.

2. Topically
Topical use of essential oils often occurs by rubbing the essential oil on the skin either neat (without dilution) or diluted with a fatty, vegetable oil (like coconut or olive oil).

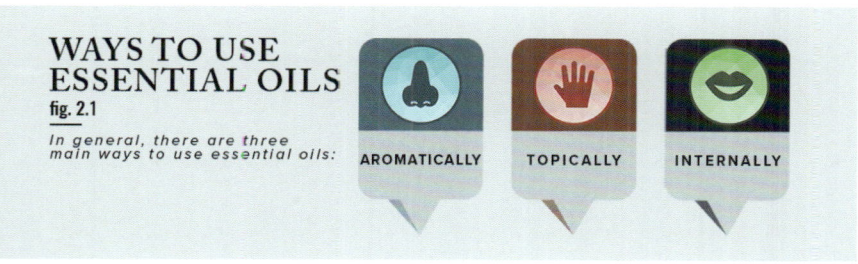

WAYS TO USE
ESSENTIAL OILS
fig. 2.1

In general, there are three main ways to use essential oils:

AROMATICALLY   TOPICALLY   INTERNALLY

3. Internally

Internal use of essential oils consists of consuming orally an essential oil deemed safe in water, food, or other drink, in a capsule diluted with a vegetable oil, or directly under the tongue. Internal use also could consist of the oil used (especially in a gel capsule) in any orifice of the body except the eyes or ears.

The molecules of essential oils are minuscule and rapidly absorbed in the body. Though they can have similar chemical components to some medications, essential oils are completely different and can't be outsmarted by bacteria and viruses like many synthetic compounds. Essential oils are able to cross the blood-brain barrier and as a result, they can often help with mental and emotional conditions.

Adulterated essential oils won't display the same pharmacological or aesthetic qualities of the natural, pure essential oils. Though the safety of an essential oil is difficult to predict from merely examining its chemical composition, in general, pure, unadulterated essential oils are very safe for use. They are usually more potent than dried herbs and could be considered "nootropics" (substances that can enhance learning, memory, and recall without other effects on the central nervous system).

Essential oils are complex natural mixtures that can vary in their chemical compositions. A typical essential oil can contain, on average, between 20 and 50 various constituents at different concentrations, which in general, can be classified into two major groups: the terpenoids and the phenylpropanoids (or aromatic compounds).

Knowing the constituents of the essential oil is important for understanding how it can work. Unlike static Lego blocks, essential oils are constantly adapting and changing and often have crossover properties. Even though a certain oil might have "better" building blocks for a particular condition doesn't mean you can only use that particular oil. Most essential oils can serve similar useful purposes, even if it wasn't the original or highest intention.

UNDERSTANDING THE STRUCTURE

Our **NERVOUS SYSTEM** is subdivided into: the central nervous system (everything inside of the head) and the peripheral nervous system (everything outside of the head). The CNS is housed in the skull and vertebral column and comprised of two parts: the brain and the spinal cord. The brain then is made of three parts: the cerebrum ("the big brain"), the cerebellum ("the little brain"), and the brainstem.

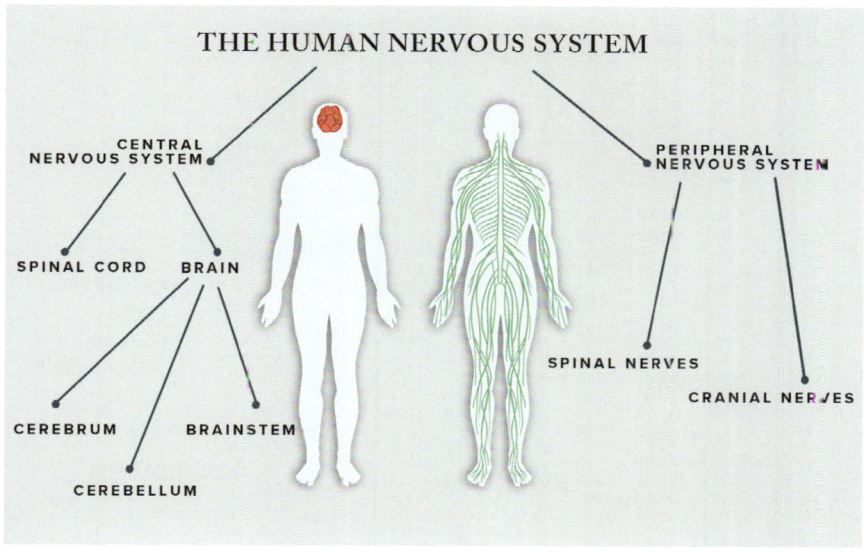

THE HUMAN NERVOUS SYSTEM

The **CEREBRUM** is the largest part of the brain and is affectionately known as "the big brain". It is divided into two halves (the right and left hemispheres) and contains five lobes: the frontal, temporal, parietal, occipital, and limbic lobes. The cerebrum, if examined from top to bottom, is defined by two distinct layers cortical and subcortical. The cortex is built by collections of neuronal cells (collectively known as grey matter) arranged in anywhere from four to six layers that are wired into networks and circuits. The cortex is folded around subcortical regions, which are organized in clumps of neurons (i.e. the amygdala is an example of a subcortical structure).

Each lobe of the brain is responsible for specific functions.

The **FRONTAL LOBE** is the most anterior—or at the front of your brain. It is responsible for motor, premotor, and supplementary motor functions. It's an extensive executive control or the "boss", responsible for regulating emotion, decision making, judgment, abstract thinking, and working memory, among other things.

The **TEMPORAL LOBE** sits below the Frontal lobe and is the lowest lobe in terms of location in the brain. The Temporal lobes contain areas that are in charge of the auditory cortex that processes sounds and speech, processing of odors, parts of the limbic system including the amygdala, hippocampus, and the parahippocampal gyrus, which we'll come back to later.

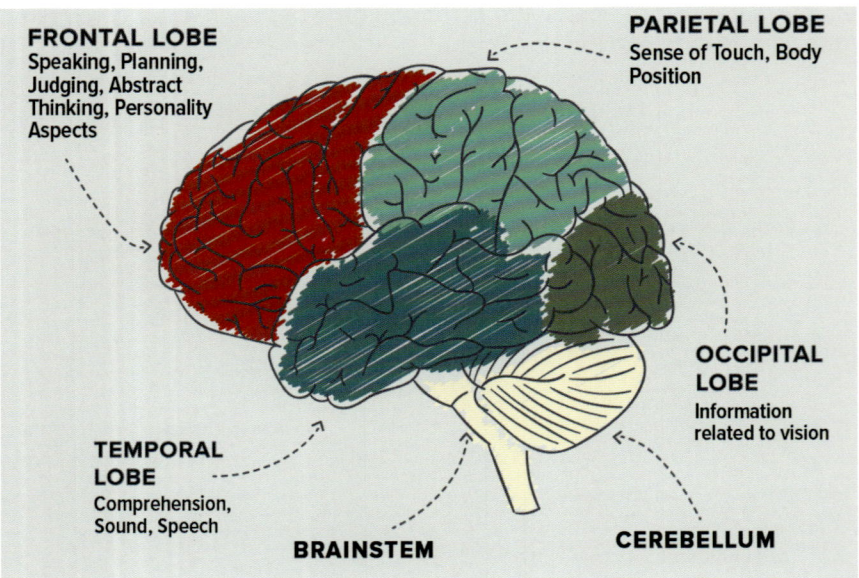

FRONTAL LOBE
Speaking, Planning, Judging, Abstract Thinking, Personality Aspects

PARIETAL LOBE
Sense of Touch, Body Position

OCCIPITAL LOBE
Information related to vision

TEMPORAL LOBE
Comprehension, Sound, Speech

BRAINSTEM

CEREBELLUM

The **PARIETAL LOBE** is surrounded by the Frontal, Temporal, and Occipital lobes and is responsible for things such as processing touch sensations and complex actions associated with spatial orientation and perception.

The **OCCIPITAL LOBE** is the furthest back and is primarily responsible for processing visual input.

The **LIMBIC LOBE** is actually constructed of various individual parts, but is often referred to as the fifth lobe. Nestled in the center of the brain, this lobe primarily includes the cingulate gyrus, the parahippocampal gyrus, the amygdala, the hippocampus, the hypothalamus, and the pineal gland. The other four lobes are visible by looking at the surface of the grey matter of the brain. However, the Limbic Lobe is hidden from plain sight, underneath the other lobes.

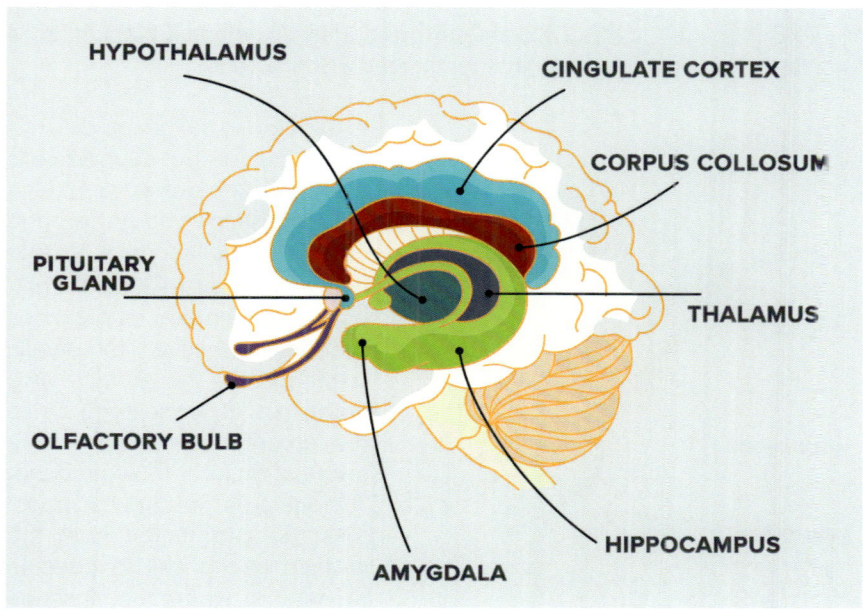

Contained between the lobes and the brainstem is the subcortical "in-between brain" known as the diencephalon, comprising less than 2 percent of the total mass of the brain and contains the pineal gland, thalamus, hypothalamus, and optic nerve, among other structures.

The **CEREBELLUM** comprises only 10 percent of the mass of the brain, but it is densely packed and highly important as it's extensively responsible for processing sensory information (including regulating equilibrium, maintaining muscle tone and postural control, and coordination of voluntary movements).

The **BRAINSTEM** is responsible for conveying information to and from the cerebrum as well as performing some special functions of its own.

The Central Nervous System (CNS) functions on two main types of cells: **NEURONS** and **GLIA**. Neurons are electrically active nerve cells that serve to convey information in the brain and nervous system through a combination of electrical and chemical signaling mechanisms. Most neurons are multipolar, meaning they consist of one cell body, dendrites that receive incoming information, and one axon that sends out information (usually in the form of neurotransmitters) through the synaptic terminals. Glia cells surround and protect neural cells like "glue". Glia cells serve many purposes including: providing support, nutrition, insulation, and helping with signal transmission between neurons. Glia cells make up about half of the mass of the brain and they are very important and underrated. Most neurons in the PNS and some in the CNS are surrounded like a "pig in a blanket" by a fatty layer known as the myelin sheath, made of glia cells.

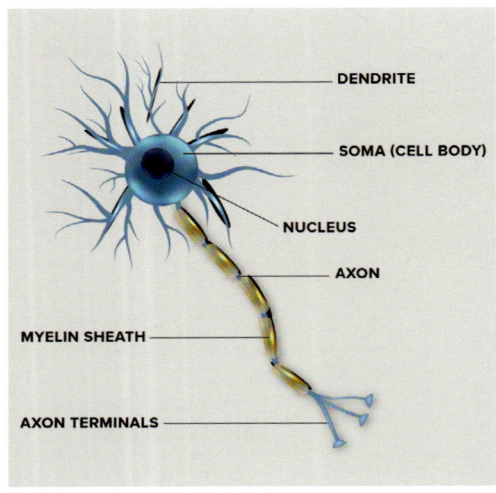

In addition to the electrical cells (neurons) and the support cells (glia), the nervous system, also influences the body through chemical messengers collectively known as **LIGANDS**, natural or manmade substances that bind selectively to specific receptors on the surface of a cell (like a "lock and key"). Once the receptor has received the information from the ligand that "unlocks" its potential, it transmits the information from the surface of the cell to deep in the interior, where the message can dramatically change the state of the cell. Ligands can communicate through cell membranes and talk to the DNA and are divided into three types: neurotransmitters, steroids, and peptides.

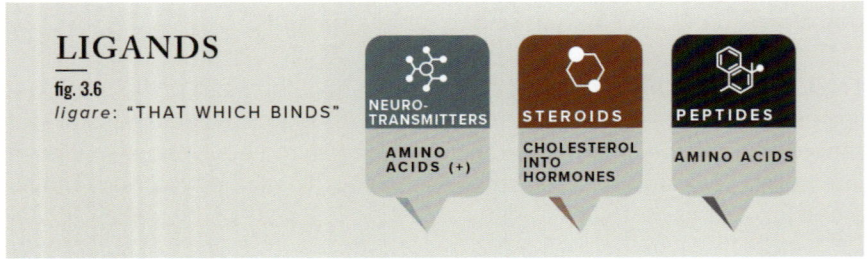

LIGANDS

fig. 3.6
ligare: "THAT WHICH BINDS"

NEURO-TRANSMITTERS	STEROIDS	PEPTIDES
AMINO ACIDS (+)	CHOLESTEROL INTO HORMONES	AMINO ACIDS

Moment by moment, the brain is sending electrical and chemical signals like seeds being planted in the soil. When a thought is formed, if a signal is strong enough, it will excite the neuron, travel along the neuron until it reaches the next neuron and then it excites that neuron and it fires. It's one giant game of telephone. With each thought, thousands of neurons may be firing at the same time and each time they are activated, they are firing together in a network. **By thinking and choosing, the landscape of the brain is redesigned so whatever you think about most will grow—literally.**

Each time a neuron connects with another neuron by sending changes and starting a new action potential causing neurons to be "wired" together, changes in the structure or function of the nervous system is happening. Changes in the synapses may strengthen and increase, or weaken and decrease the number of connections between neurons. Neurons aren't just creating their own individual pathways, but also huge networks of connections. This ability for the brain to change over time is what science calls:

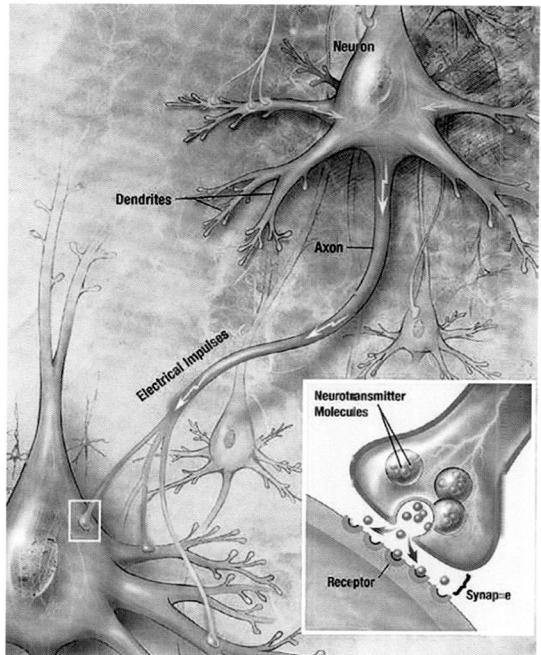

NEUROPLASTICITY.
Neuroplasticity is the natural result of each sensory input, motor act, association, reward signal, action plan, or awareness that feeds the mind. Behavior will lead to changes in how the brain wires and fires, just as changes in brain circuitry will lead to behavioral modifications.

Unlike the other senses, olfaction stands alone as the ONLY sensory input that doesn't have to go through the thalamus in the brainstem before being processed by the brain. The neurons in the olfactory system have direct access to the brain and are the only part of the brain exposed to the outside world. There are two theories as to how the brain perceives odor molecules as the specific odorant: shape pattern theory and vibrational theory. Shape pattern theory claims that the olfactory receptor is activated because the molecules of the odorant "fit" into the shape of the receptor that best corresponds to the shape of the odorant like a key fitting into a lock. With vibration theory, the olfactory sensory neurons are activated chiefly from the vibrational frequency of the odor molecules.

Both shape-pattern theory and vibration theory can be useful in the context of essential oils and fit the models of chemistry and quantum physics (respectively). Regardless of the theory, evidence exists that we detect odors based on the pattern of activity (either chemical or vibrational) across various receptor types. The intensity of an odor will change depending on the activation of the receptors, which is why weak and strong concentrations of odorants don't smell quite the same. This explains why diffusing pepper-mint essential oil may have a different perceived scent than directly inhaling it from the bottle.

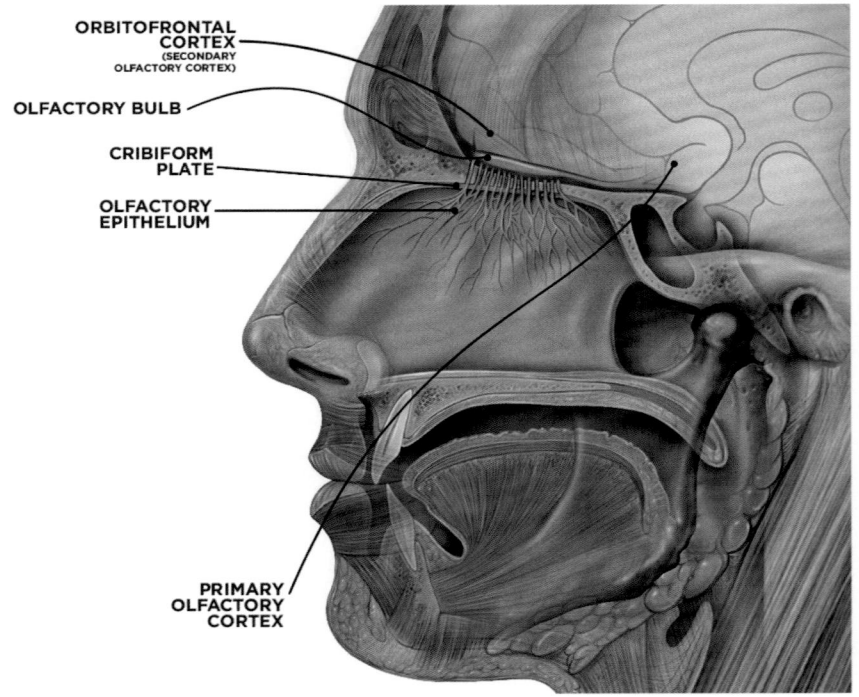

ORBITOFRONTAL CORTEX
(SECONDARY OLFACTORY CORTEX)

OLFACTORY BULB

CRIBIFORM PLATE

OLFACTORY EPITHELIUM

PRIMARY OLFACTORY CORTEX

Because the only exposed part of the brain to the outside world sits at the top of the nasal cavity, both passive and direct inhalation is a powerful way to use essential oils. Whether aromatically, topically, or through ingestion, essential oils have the ability to cross the blood-brain barrier because they are lipid soluble and under 500 amu in weight.

SUPPORTING THE STRUCTURE

Many functional issues in the mind and body are actually a result of structural deficiencies. Countless research studies in the ast few decades have repeatedly shown the interaction between the introduction of substances (such as vitamins, minerals, and amino acids through food) to influence the structure and function of the brain in positive ways.

DIET

In short, the brain is fueled by two main things: glucose and oxygen. These are the absolute basic requirements for energy, development, and survival. A typical brain uses about 10 percent of the oxygen needed for the body and a whopping 50 to 60 percent of the glucose consumed, so if you ever feel like you're starving, it's because your neurons and glia literally are starving. In general, a good balance of complex carbohydrates, quality protein sources, and healthy fats are the best way to serve your brain optimal nutrition.

EXERCISE

Exercise is another key factor for keeping your brain in optimum shape. Once again, depending on which school of thought you ascribe to, the type, frequency and intensity of exercise that is "best" will be highly variable. Similarly to the approach to a healthy diet, the "best" form of exercise is the one that is best suited for your body. Your brain thrives on exercise for a couple of key reasons: increased oxygen and blood flow and decreased stress response. The increased blood flow doesn't just affect the brain in the moment, it actually has long term benefit, too. Exercise may have a direct affect on the brain's ability to fight aging. Though the hippocampus specifically responds well to aerobic exercise, various parts of the brain, including the prefrontal cortex and other cortical regions can be greatly affected by even 30 minutes of daily brisk walking. Multiple well-controlled studies in children, adults, and the elderly have shown not just the impact of exercise on memory and learning, but on executive function and decision making.

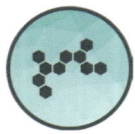

AMINO ACIDS

Amino acids, the building blocks of proteins, are key for forming and maintaining components in our brains and bodies, including neurotransmitters. There are nine "essential" amino acids that must be consumed daily in order to support survival and because they cannot be created by the body, they must be consumed through food sources or supplementation. The other 11 amino acids are considered "conditionally essential" and the body will produce them if they're not consumed through dietary means. Amino acids are absorbed quickly into the brain and body network and if consumed in their free (predigested) form, can be effectively taken orally and do not need digestive enzymes in order to work.

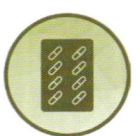

VITAMINS

Without vitamins, we suffer less than vibrant existences, as vitamins assist in regulating metabolism and the biochemical process that releases energy from digested food. Vitamins are considered micronutrients because they are needed in much smaller quantities when compared to nutrients such as carbohydrates, proteins, fats, and water. Some vitamins are water-soluble and others dissolve in oil and both kinds are needed for proper functioning in the body. The water-soluble vitamins (such as vitamin C and the B-complex vitamins) must be consumed daily as the body cannot store and thus excretes them within hours. Oil-soluble vitamins (such as vitamins A, D, E, and K) can be stored for longer periods of time in the body's fatty tissue and the liver.

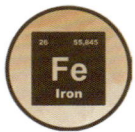

MINERALS + TRACE ELEMENTS

Most of us are walking around with mineral deficiencies and we don't even realize it. Thanks to overly processed food and nutrient-depleted soil where our food is harvested from, our bodies are not absorbing the minerals and trace elements necessary for proper brain function. Of the 44 minerals and trace elements that can be found in the ocean, over 20 of those have disappeared from the land and fertilizers added to the soil are further depleting our minerals. Just as is the case with both amino acid and vitamin deficiencies, lack of proper minerals can result in emotional symptoms.

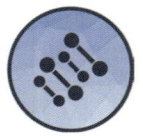

ESSENTIAL FATTY ACIDS

Nearly two-thirds of the mass of the brain is comprised of fat. Not only are glia cells primarily comprised of fat (known as the white matter of the brain), but the signal transmission in the central and peripheral nervous system is dependent on fat for proper functioning. Consuming healthy fats, including omega-3 and omega-6 essential fatty acids, supports proper brain function. There are both vegetarian and non-vegetarian sources of omega-3 and omega-6 fatty acids, but the important thing is to get a lot of them and get them regularly. There are two essential fatty acids, both polyunsaturated fats: linoleic acid (LA) is the precursor to omega-6 fatty acid, and alpha-linoleic acid (ALA) is the precursor to omega-3 fatty acid. Humans cannot synthesize essential fatty acids, so they must be consumed through diet to prevent deficiency. Omega-3 fatty acids play important roles in vision, nervous system function, immune and inflammatory responses, and modulation of gene expression.

ANTIOXIDANTS

Antioxidants serve the body by slowing the natural oxidation process that causes aging. Because brain cell membranes are the most susceptible to lipid peroxidation (from exposure to sources like paint, cigarette smoke, gasoline, cleaning fluids, and chemicals of all kinds), antioxidants fight the free radical damage and protect the cells and nerves from damage.

ENZYMES

Enzymes are energized protein molecules and they play a necessary role in virtually all of the biochemical activities in the body including digesting food, stimulating the brain, providing cellular energy, and repairing tissues, organs, and cells. The body manufactures a supply of enzymes, but it can and should also obtain supplementation of enzymes through food. Sadly, due to processed and highly cooked food, many of our bodies are suffering the ability to make enough enzymes to compensate and further supplementation is needed. The majority of commercially available enzymes are digestive enzymes from various sources and are typically available over the counter in tablet, capsule, powder, and liquid forms. For maximum benefit, any digestive enzyme supplement you take should contain all of the major enzyme groups: amylase, protease, and lipase.

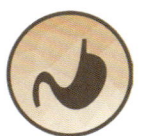

THE GUT/BRAIN CONNECTION

Research is increasingly showing that many physical and emotional conditions are greatly affected and/or relieved by the digestive tract. In fact, 75 percent of your serotonin receptors are in your gut. This is important because serotonin helps in mood regulation and low serotonin levels have been associated with feelings of depression. Taking a high-potency probiotic to support gut health boosts the brain and body's ability to combat stress and illness.

Understanding that we are more than just the brains that are in our bodies and the things we're consuming (or applying) to affect it is key to improving our bodies and minds. What we put in our bodies affects the expression of our minds. Setting the foundation with practicals like diet, exercise, and healthy supplementation provides us with a strong edifice from which we can express our lives to the world around us.

UNDERSTANDING THE FUNCTION

The biological, neurochemical, and metaphysical functions of our bodies (the hardware) operate on the software of our soul (our mind, will and emotions). The functions of the "soul" (mind, will, and emotions) include the cognitive functions (or "cognitive processes"): perception (or alertness), attention, cognition, memory, emotional regulation, language, motor skills, visual and spatial processing, and executive function.

Five principles are true for all brains:
1. The cognitive processes are active, rather than passive.
2. The cognitive processes are remarkably efficient and accurate.
3. The cognitive processes handle positive information better than negative information.
4. The cognitive processes are interrelated with one another; they do not operate in isolation.
5. Many cognitive processes rely on both bottom-up and top-down processing.

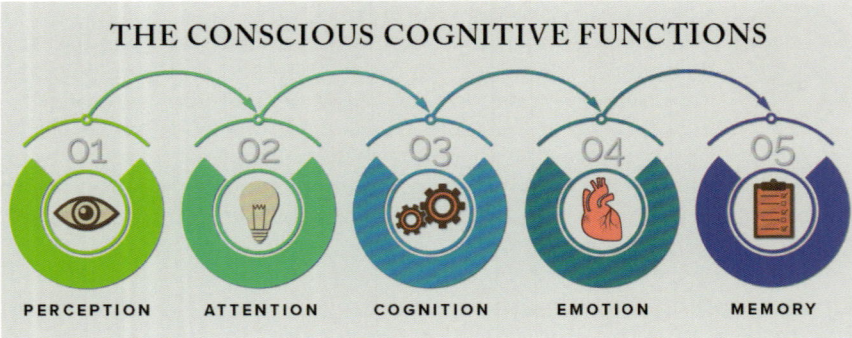

THE CONSCIOUS COGNITIVE FUNCTIONS

01 PERCEPTION 02 ATTENTION 03 COGNITION 04 EMOTION 05 MEMORY

The main difference between conscious cognition and unconscious cognition is simply the amount of neural firing or neuropeptides at work at a given time. The more intense or prolonged the neural network fires, the more a cognition will rise from the unconscious and into the conscious. In our working model, we reduce the conscious cognitive functions that combines the mind, will, and emotions into one linear order (though they are happening usually simultaneously and not necessarily in succession): perception, attention, cognition, memory, and emotional regulation. They are understood as the functions operating on the structure of the brain and may manifest as "mind," "will," or "emotion" as the expression.

The brain is designed to naturally change over time through neuro-plasticity. Age affects the level of neuroplasticity as does trauma. By and large, throughout life, neurons are constantly shifting and changing depending on what stimuli and thoughts the individual attends to.

We don't see the world as it is, but rather we see it filtered through our sensory systems. We cannot separate perception from memory or from cognition. As soon as you perceive something, it's in your memory. We see a view of the world that's constructed and stored in our memory by the brain. Memory is often not accurate to the specific events, but rather it has been filtered through our sensory systems and perceptual biases. Most of the processing of the world comes from both a "top-down" and a "bottom-up" approach (the brain's ability to perceive the object [top-down] from the senses [bottom-up]). **The brain relies on both the sensory input and the perceptual cues in order to make sense of almost every scenario in life. In a neurotypical brain that isn't suffering from cognitive stress, trauma, or abnormal environmental influences, this is going to be a relatively simplistic and rapid process.**

As we live, we build experiences, memories, and associations around what we have learned over time and our brains begin to create "shortcuts" to streamline the amount of time it takes to perceive data and process it. Because our brains are wired to make associations rapidly, the brain will look for as many "shortcuts" to the perception as possible (known as "heuristics"). Our knowledge of what is going on around us then feeds into what we perceive about the world. Our expectations—the heuristics our brain creates—feed into what we then perceive through our senses.

With each of the senses, with the exception of olfaction, most sensory information is processed similarly and passes through the brain stem before localizing in the specific association cortices. There are three distinct phases that start at the neural and chemical level before gathering and being processed and forming the cognitive functions. When a sensory stimulus comes in through one of the senses, your brain is alerted to it and if you give it attention, the perception of the stimuli will continue. The attention then gives way to cognition—the conscious mental processing of the stimulus. The more something is attended to and cognitively processed, it will then be stored in short-term memory and potentially in long-term memory. The likelihood of a stimulus being stored in the memory system will be even greater if it is linked to an emotion.

Humans are designed to withstand stress, and in reality, not all stress is bad. There are two types of stress, one positive and one negative: eustress (positive) and distress (negative). Eustress is a form of positive stress that motivates, allows you to focus energy and achieve. Distress (or simply "stress") comes as a result of a stressor—an internal or external event or stimulus that interrupts equilibrium and prompts a response. Unresolved stress not only affects our brains, but it can be damaging to our bodies. According to a study from the American Medical Association, 75 percent of all illnesses and diseases people suffer from today have stress as a clear factor. Dr. Caroline Leaf argues that 75 to 98 percent of mental and physical illnesses come from one's thought life and stress plays a huge role.

Stressors are sure to come throughout life. The variable in question is not if or when stressors will happen, but how we will respond. Two individuals can experience the same stressor in very different ways. Their response will be based primarily in how they have responded to stressors in the past. Naturally, the brain wants to make work as easy as possible so it begins to automate information—memories, emotions, thoughts—that are stored in the unconscious mind (metacognitive) and only are accessed when they're needed.

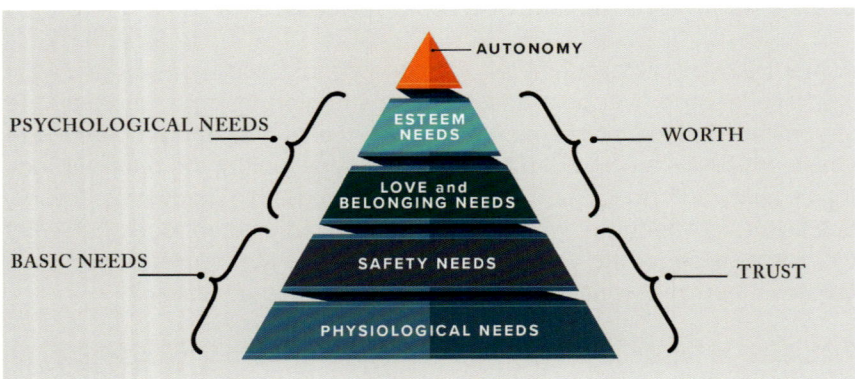

Data shows that up to 99 percent of the decisions you make are based on what you have built and automatized into your unconscious, metacognitive level. There are a few fundamental needs, that if met, will create a security that enables an individual to exist with resilience to stress and openness. These needs can build upon one another, but also can dynamically innervate to create a "whole" and balanced individual. Humans are wired for connection (a.k.a. attachment, love, or belonging). The hierarchy of needs defines the ideal conditions in which autonomy, built on trust and worth, can be achieved.

The autonomy of an individual is built on two primary forces: trust and worth. Physiological needs and security needs combine to form trust, which affirms to the individual that their basic needs will be met in a timely and consistent manner. Psychological needs such as belonging and esteem combine to form worth, which involves the individual understanding that they are worthy of giving and receiving affirmation and affection. If there is a breach in trust or a lack of understanding of worth, the individual may feel a level of vulnerability that acts as an internal stress. The vulnerability itself is not alarming, but is a gateway either into positive or negative emotions depending on the response of the person.

Stress—internal or external—affects our perceived level of vulnerability but even more influential is the effect of trauma on an individual's ability to respond properly to stimuli and employ resiliency in the face of vulnerability. Trauma happens when a stressor is either so severe, is repeated consistently, or happens for a prolonged period of time that the individual is not equipped to respond or it feels too overwhelming. Traumatic stress tends to evoke two emotional extremes: feeling either too much (overwhelmed) or too little (numb) emotion. The types of trauma can vary, but may include violence (community, domestic, school), early childhood trauma, medical trauma, natural disasters, neglect, abuse (physical, sexual, emotional, or verbal), terrorism, and traumatic grief. In general, we classify trauma into three types: Trauma A (neglect), Trauma B (abuse), and Complex Trauma.

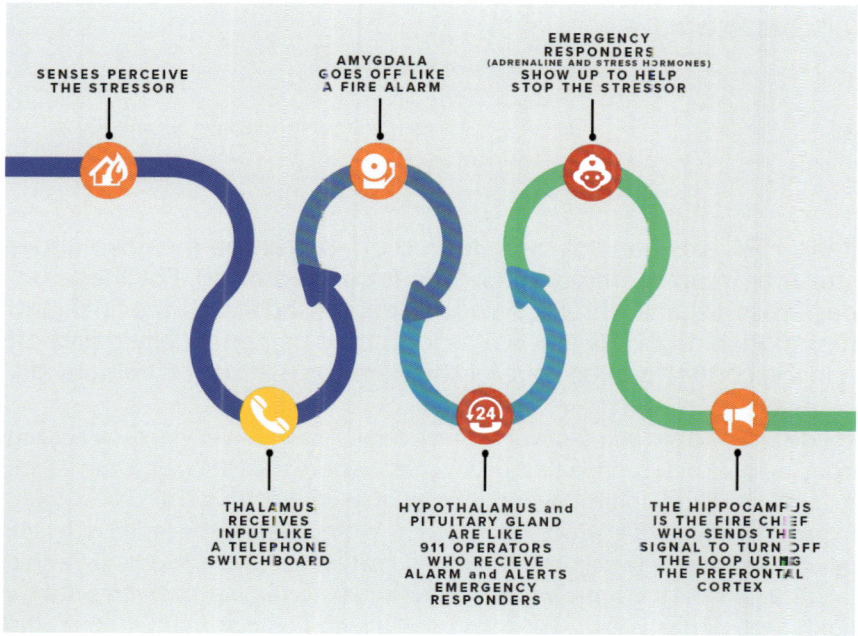

SENSES PERCEIVE THE STRESSOR

AMYGDALA GOES OFF LIKE A FIRE ALARM

EMERGENCY RESPONDERS (ADRENALINE AND STRESS HORMONES) SHOW UP TO HELP STOP THE STRESSOR

THALAMUS RECEIVES INPUT LIKE A TELEPHONE SWITCHBOARD

HYPOTHALAMUS and PITUITARY GLAND ARE LIKE 911 OPERATORS WHO RECIEVE ALARM and ALERTS EMERGENCY RESPONDERS

THE HIPPOCAMPUS IS THE FIRE CHIEF WHO SENDS THE SIGNAL TO TURN OFF THE LOOP USING THE PREFRONTAL CORTEX

When the brain is stressed or suffering from trauma, two types of responses are formed to combat the stressor: the Hypothalamic-Pituitary-Adrenal axis (HPA axis) and the immune system.

It is the job of the nervous system to monitor the environment, assess the situation, interpret the signals, and organize the appropriate responses in the body. The HPA axis responds to external threats and the immune system responds to threats internally (like viruses or bacteria). When the HPA axis is engaged and mobilizing the body, the work of the immune system is suppressed in order to conserve energy. When the HPA axis has completed its loop and is shut off, the immune system function is restored.

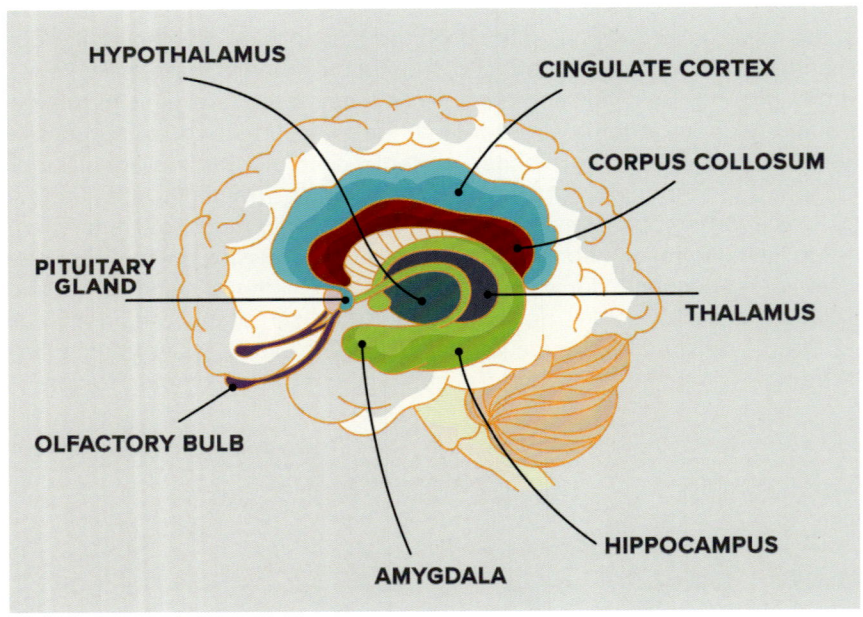

HYPOTHALAMUS

CINGULATE CORTEX

CORPUS COLLOSUM

PITUITARY GLAND

THALAMUS

OLFACTORY BULB

HIPPOCAMPUS

AMYGDALA

If the HPA axis has not been turned off (as can be the case under stress or trauma), immune function is compromised. For those under stress, trauma, chronic pain, or in depressed states, the fire alarm that triggers the HPA axis stress loop may be continually going off and the control loop be severely hindered to not turn off without aid.

Those who are slow to recover from adversity, have fewer signals traveling from the prefrontal cortex to the amygdala, where the HPA axis is turned on and off. A lack of control over the emotional control loop (HPA axis) could happen because of a structural issue (i.e. brain injury) or because of a lack of connections between the prefrontal cortex and the amygdala. People with trauma have issues with their prefrontal cortex not shutting off their emotional alarms. They live in constant flight, fight, or freeze. When the connection between the prefrontal cortex and the amygdala is strengthened, resiliency increases.

Essential oils aid the brain and body by supporting the immune system as well as reducing strain on the brain when under stress or trauma. Properties in some essential oils have been found to modulate the hypothalamic–pituitary–adrenal (HPA) axis and influence hippocampal gene expression, helping to turn off the fire alarm when it is blaring and increasing effectiveness in all other cognitive functions, including perception, attention, cognition, memory, and emotional regulation.

YOUR MOM'S BRAIN

We all inherit DNA from our parents, but now science shows us that other factors can be passed down such as memories, emotions, stress, and even trauma. The science of epigenetics gives us an explanation for sometimes why we feel the way we do and how things can be imprinted on our subconscious mind.

Epigenetics explains the regulation of gene expression that is not based on DNA sequence but, rather, is controlled by heritable and potentially reversible changes to the DNA by way of methylation or modification to the chromatin structure.

Not only can genetic modification of the DNA affect our lives, the epigenetic markers can also play a role in how our genes are expressed. In order for cells to operate "correctly," both the DNA sequence and the epigenetic factors must be normal. People who have epigenetic misregulation may suffer from a disease or condition, even if their DNA sequences are functionally impeccable with no disease mutations or pre-disposing DNA sequence variants. Traumatic memories and stress are being shown to pass from one generation to another. The transmission of the unconscious mind may continue beyond the second generation and also include the grandchildren, great-grandchildren and perhaps others as well and is known as the transgenerational transmission of trauma.

The traditional definition of epigenetics is the study of heritable changes in gene expression that are not due to changes in the underlying DNA sequence. The coating on the DNA sequence becomes a sort of "memory" of the cell and since all cells in our body carry this kind of memory, it becomes a constant physical reminder of past events, our own and those of our parents, grandparents and beyond. It's as though the body is keeping the score.

What part of who we are is a result of our genetics and what part is a result of the environment we've grown up in and around? A traditional ratio for "nature versus nurture" is 60 percent of who you are is a result of your genetics and 40 percent has to do with your upbringing. However, what we can see from the study of epigenetics is that just because you have the genetic propensity doesn't mean those genes will be turned on (what is also known as the genes being "expressed"). Our thoughts, even our imaginations can get "under the skin" of our DNA and can turn certain genes on and certain genes off, changing the structure of the neural pathways in the brain. The ability to switch on or off our genetic expression can have profound effect on our brains and bodies.

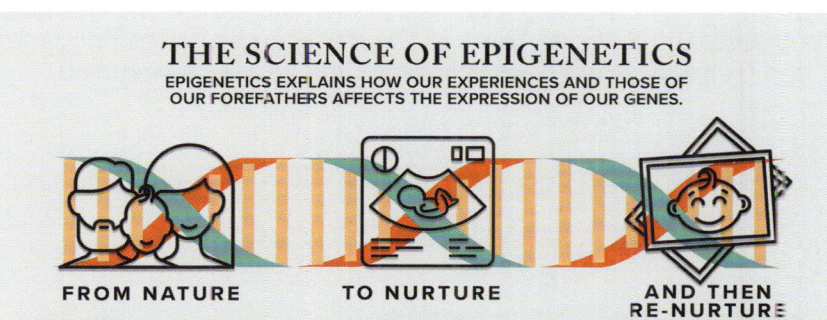

THE SCIENCE OF EPIGENETICS

EPIGENETICS EXPLAINS HOW OUR EXPERIENCES AND THOSE OF OUR FOREFATHERS AFFECTS THE EXPRESSION OF OUR GENES.

FROM NATURE

Genes passed down from our father and mother act as a set of instructions for our cells and influence what we look like on the outside and how we work on the inside.

The genes children inherit from their biological parents provide information that guides their development. For example, how tall they could eventually become or the kind of temperament they could have.

TO NURTURE

During development, the DNA that makes up our genes accumulates chemical marks that determine how much or little of the genes is expressed.

This collection of chemical marks is known as the "epigenome." When experiences during development rearrange the epigenetic marks that govern gene expression, they can change whether and how genes release the information they carry.

This explains why genetically identical twins can exhibit different behaviors, skills, health, and achievement.

AND THEN RE-NURTURE

The epigenome can be affected by positive experiences, such as supportive relationships and opportunities for learning, or negative influences, such as environmental toxins or stressful life circumstances.

These experiences—positive or negative—leave a unique epigenetic "signature" on the genes. These signatures can be temporary or permanent and both types affect how easily the genes are switched on or off.

Young brains are particularly sensitive to epigenetic changes. However, science shows how positive input throughout life can change the expression of genes and epigenomes.

Trust and worth, the elements necessary for a healthy autonomous individual, aren't just needed when you're a small child who can talk or walk or play. Rather, the process of learning trust and worth begins before your conscious mind is fully developed. The epigenetic expression of your genes begins adapting before you even are aware of the world around you. Not only can the epigenetic markers be present on our genes because of our forefathers, but our time in the womb and as newborn babies profoundly affects how our brains respond to stress, trauma, and establish resiliency in the world. Recent research now shows that the more maternal care received following birth, the better the individual's resiliency in response to stress is later in life.

In short, though a person may have experienced stress or trauma before or after birth and it has caused epigenetic changes to their DNA, they are not without hope of change. Each cognitive function—every thought, feeling, or memory—we engage in, whether consciously or unconsciously, sends an electrical or chemical signal to our body that can change the expression of our genes and alter each cell in our body.

The universal law of "sowing and reaping" exists whether you believe in it or not, just like gravity is not predicated on our agreement. Sowing and reaping says that whatever seed you put into the ground will produce a fruit according to its kind. Time is a huge factor in the process of sowing and reaping. **In our minds and bodies, most of the memories, decisions, thoughts, and words sown are not "harvested" back in life until days, weeks, months, or years later. In fact, the choices our parents and grandparents made "back in the day" can be passed down to us and "reaped" in our lives years after the incidents occurred.**

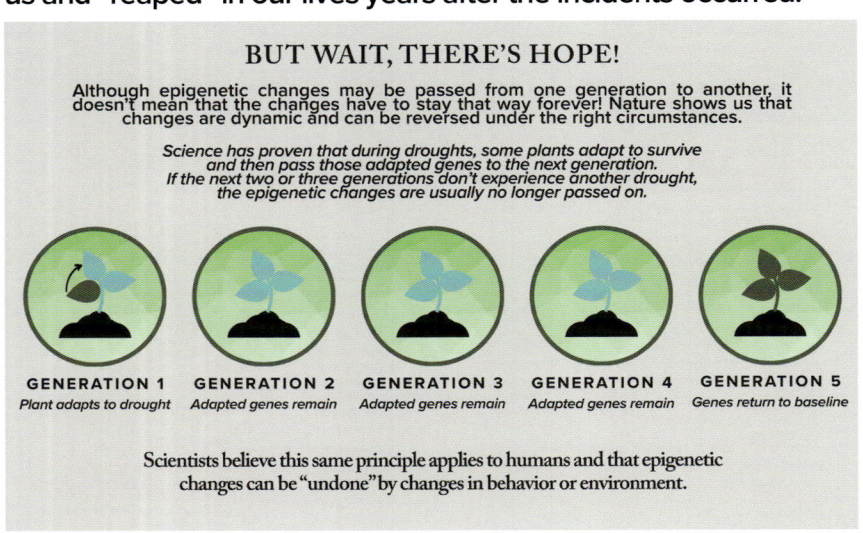

BUT WAIT, THERE'S HOPE!

Although epigenetic changes may be passed from one generation to another, it doesn't mean that the changes have to stay that way forever! Nature shows us that changes are dynamic and can be reversed under the right circumstances.

Science has proven that during droughts, some plants adapt to survive and then pass those adapted genes to the next generation. If the next two or three generations don't experience another drought, the epigenetic changes are usually no longer passed on.

GENERATION 1	GENERATION 2	GENERATION 3	GENERATION 4	GENERATION 5
Plant adapts to drought	*Adapted genes remain*	*Adapted genes remain*	*Adapted genes remain*	*Genes return to baseline*

Scientists believe this same principle applies to humans and that epigenetic changes can be "undone" by changes in behavior or environment.

It might not seem fair that we carry around the seeds sown by our forefathers, but the wonderful thing is that we don't have to live with their negative effects. The universal law of sowing and reaping was designed to bring favorable outcomes if good seed is sown correctly. We can reap the good or the bad from the choices of not just our lives, but those who went before us. But just because the epigenetic change has been "sown" or marked on our DNA, doesn't mean that we have to live with it forever.

You may have received all of the right nutrients—physically, emotionally, spiritually—from the time before you were born, through your infancy and childhood and to the present. However, the reality for most people is that they carry unresolved, repressed or expressed epigenetic markers from both of their parents, their parents' parents, their parents' parents' parents and others. It can be easy to continue carrying the weight of all that happened to you up to this point, but it's important to not just let go of the trauma, but to forgive and let go of those who failed to give you what you needed or desired. This act of release of others allows us to walk forward into freedom in a new way. It is nature and nurture and re-nurture.

SUPPORTING THE FUNCTION

Odors are powerful for awaking memories partly because of their direct access to the neural substrates of olfaction, emotion, associative learning, and memory. Memories that are triggered by scent are known as "Proustian memories" and differ from semantic memory (information storage) and other types of episodic memory (storage of specific events). Proustian memories aren't triggered by the same cues (like visual and verbal). Odors elicit more affective, old, rare, and evocative personal memories.

Since essential oils are aromatic compounds, they naturally can have a profound effect on the ability to retrieve memories and prompt emotions. But how else can they help the brain? The chemical compounds of essential oils can affect the brain and body in our five main cognitive functions: perception, attention, cognition, memory, and emotional regulation.

Just like essential oils are created to help balance the plant, they also can have profound affect on our cells and even fill in the gaps where we need a little extra balancing.

Chemically, essential oils can act on our cells in a few distinct ways:
1. They engage in selective binding with specific molecular targets such as neuro- or hormone receptors. Human hormones and neurotransmitters are nearly identical in molecular structure to those produced in plants. This fact is not only astounding, but it provides amazing hope for the ability to change our brain chemistry simply by using the secondary metabolites of essential oils.

2. They non-selectively cause a disturbance of the three-dimensional structure of proteins (known as protein conformation).

3. They bond covalently to DNA and RNA, modifying gene expression. Thanks to essential oils, the ability to modify how our genes are expressed is possible due to the same covalent and non-covalent modifications of proteins.

4. They change membrane permeability and the function of membrane proteins. Essential oils can change the permeability of membranes. Most water-soluble mol-

ecules cannot penetrate cell membranes, only non-polar or very small molecules (like oxygen, carbon dioxide, or water) can get through uninhibited. Inside the cell membrane is where all of the activity of the cell takes place like the necessary exchanges of amino acids, sugar, and signaling—all controlled by proteins integrated in the membrane.

Not only can essential oils affect the cell membranes, but that is where the work of changing the DNA and RNA of the cell actually begins. One simple theory on how essential oils work at the cellular level in our brains and bodies is known as PSM Paradigm. PSM stands for three different chemical component types contained in some essential oils (or can be mixed in a custom blend) that speed cellular healing: phenols (or phenyl-propanoids), sesquiterpenes, and monoterpenes. This chemical combination in a single oil or layering of multiple oils high in these three compounds helps to explain how a single anointment or application of essential oils is able to bring about an instant and permanent healing. First, the phenols clean the receptor sites. Then the sesquiterpenes delete bad information from cellular memory. Lastly, monoterpenes restore or awaken the correct information in the cell's memory (DNA).

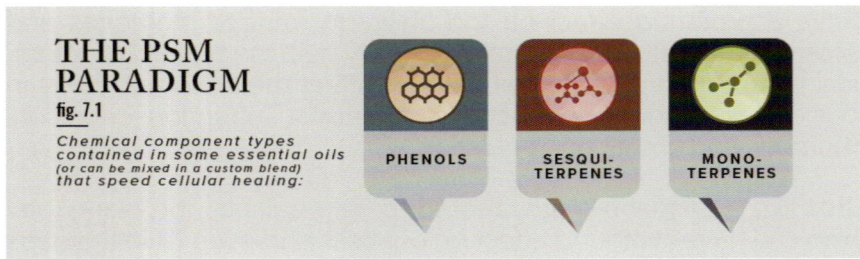

THE PSM PARADIGM
fig. 7.1
Chemical component types contained in some essential oils (or can be mixed in a custom blend) that speed cellular healing:

PHENOLS   SESQUI-TERPENES   MONO-TERPENES

The PSM paradigm—along with the other components that make up essential oils like alcohols, ketones, ethers, and esters—help to defragment the brain and allow for the chance to create lasting change at a cellular level. However, this paradigm is only one possible mechanism for how and why essential oils work so powerfully. We can also argue that electrical, magnetic, and vibrational etiologies are also explanations for the effectiveness of essential oils.

The wonderful thing about essential oils is that many of them have crossover properties chemically and can do functions because of their ability as secondary metabolites to adapt to environments. Since essential oils are extremely diverse, resilient, resourceful, and intelligent, it stands to reason that many, many more varieties of essential oils than even those covered in this chapter could be beneficial for the brain.

WHY "MIND OVER MATTER" MATTERS

According to quantum physics, matter can be both a particle and a wave. What used to be thought of as either/or can now be considered both/and.

The study of quantum mechanics was not a replacement for Newtonian (or "classical") physics, which remains valid within its limits, but rather is like flipping over the other side of the coin to discover a new face. Classical physics applies still to the large-scale world whereas the study of quantum units lies in the subatomic realm—the invisible universe underlying, embedded in, and constructing the fabric of everything around us.

Quantum physics is the study of the nature, properties, or motion of quantities of matter and energy. Quantum theory states that the universe comes in bits and pieces (quanta) and the physics or mechanics examines the study of this phenomenon.

The basic tenants of quantum physics states:
1. A most basic (subatomic) piece of matter **can** behave as either a particle or a wave without violating its status as little hunks of something.

2. The piece of matter **will** behave as either a particle _or_ a wave depending on the role of the individual and their relation to the matter.

3. Unlike classical physics that has defined predictions of the outcome, in quantum, the predicted outcome of the matter is not only infinite and variable, but can actually be influenced by the individual and their relation to the matter.

We are dealing with units of energy that exist in patterns of probability waves. It isn't to predict what will actually happen, but only to predict the probabilities of various possible results. Matter in particle form is thought to exist if/until there are potential choices to be made and then the matter takes on a wave form depending on the expectation or intended outcome.

In short, quantum physics helps us to explain:

1. How the brain functions in endlessly resilient and creative ways beyond what we can know from just examining the data and/or anatomical structure.

2. How and why directed mental effort produces systematic and predictable changes in brain function.

3. How and why essential oils can do unexpected things to/on our brains beyond their chemical components.

Quantum physics provides the "why" behind how our mind is greater than just the matter of our brains and the essential oils we use on them.

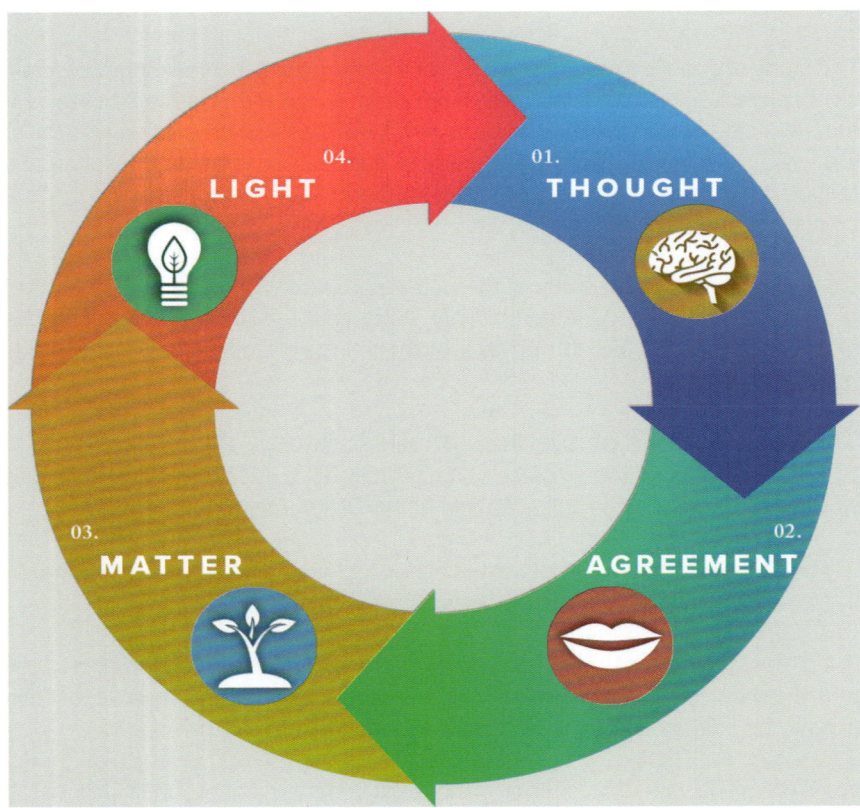

To convey how quantum physics affects the mind and brain, we defined a new model. This model works on a cyclical process beginning with the thought, adding agreement, resulting in physical matter, then the manifestation of the light (life).

Conscious thought (what we see from the data as being electrical and chemical energy) requires agreement in order to produce matter. Agreement can come in the form of a conscious attention to the thought—some call this "mindfulness", but even more powerful than just mindfulness is verbal agreement. Words are energy and energy affects (and even creates) matter. Once agreement (whether in conscious acknowledgement or verbally) has been made, the matter can exist.

Under Newtonian physics, the old question of "if a tree (the particle or wave) falls in the forest...", it will fall because the law of gravity requires it to regardless if a person is there to observe it. In the realm of quantum physics, the tree (the subatomic particle or wave) might not even be visible unless the observer is there to watch it fall. Matter can only exist in some cases when an individual is present to see it exist. There is a dependence then on the individual for the matter to exist in the first place and then their influence (through conscious choice) can allow the matter to change forms and beget new possibilities (light/life).

A new term has emerged recently, "self-directed neuroplasticity", as a general description of the principle indicating that focused training and effort can systematically alter brain function in a predictable and potentially therapeutic manner. We've discussed in detail how the brain naturally engages in neuroplasticity, but self-directed neuroplasticity gives language to the process of consciously choosing to engage in agreement in order to modify the matter of your spirit, soul, and body.

As we have seen and what has been confirmed from the data, in the molecular world, many possibilities exist and your conscious choice to agree with them or not will dictate the outcome. Some scientists say it's like a "packet of possibilities"—a yeast that acts like a catalyst on the matter changing it from one form to another. Another way of defining this is "faith". Using that term is risky as it can conjure a variety of images depending on your experience and biases. However, when I use "faith", would like to apply the definition, "the hopeful expectation of good."

The subconscious mind can be influenced by a variety of things (our spirits, memories, emotions, epigenetic expression, etc.), but it serves as the birthplace of the thoughts we then can choose to apply agreement (faith) to in order to shape and form our reality.

If there were levels of potency or speed of change or healing they would function in this order and scale according to quantum theories:
1. Neuroplasticity alone
2. Neuroplasticity (with essential oils)
3. Self-directed neuroplasticity (without essential oils)
4. Self-directed neuroplasticity (with essential oils)

We've talked previously about how the chemistry of essential oils affect the cells in our body. But quantum mechanics has another explanation: frequency. Science has shown that every living thing carries a frequency, the measurable rate of electrical energy between two points. Another way of looking at frequency is the rate at which molecules expressed as waves, vibrate. Every living thing has a frequency. Sound is a vibration. Light is a vibration. Sound molecules can travel as a wave in the air, water, or in a solid. That vibration is in every living thing and is referred to as frequency or energy.

Chemicals in our environment, bad food and water, stress, fear, negative thinking, and lack of sleep can all lower the frequencies of our bodies. A healthy body typically has a frequency between 62 and 78 MHz (megahertz). When our body dips below the normal frequency range, even to 58 MHz, sickness and diseases can begin. Royal Raymond Rife, one of the early researchers of frequency, said that every disease has its own frequency and a substance with a higher frequency will alter the disease with the lower frequency. The great news is that essential oils range in frequency from 52 MHz all the way up to Rose, which has a frequency of 320 MHz. When we use and diffuse essential oils we are raising our frequency and strengthening our bodies and brains.

Instead of saying what an essential oil *will* do or what issues it *will* address, rather the manifestation of the potential of the oil is dependent on the hopeful expectation of good (faith) of the user.

Therefore, based on the data and according to our model, the most advantageous and fastest way to change both the structure and function of your brain and your body is to engage first in self-directed neuroplasticity (agreement in your mind) and state verbally the expected outcome while using essential oils (aromatically, topically, or internally). This combination of multi-frequency agreement (i.e. sound and light) engages the thought with intention to manifest matter and form the light of new possibilities in your life and world.

DOORS:
HEALING THE MIND

As you embark on a journey of inner healing in spirit, soul, and body, you'll discover that there are doors you never knew existed. Sometimes you find the doorway and open it to discover there are glorious secrets and brilliant thoughts on the other side But more often than not, those doors have been sealed by trauma nestled deep in the subconscious and opening them reveals dank, dark rooms. As you open the door, there's no need to be afraid of what you find. You just need to bring in the light. Go into every room with light

and see what needs to be cleaned. Your mind will become new as you illuminate the newly discovered parts that used to be closed to the world.

If our cognitive functions are like seeds planted in our minds, then toxic thoughts, stress, trauma, epigenetic markers negatively expressed could all be like weeds polluting our crop. In regards to essential oils and inner healing, we're not talking about mind erasing where you apply an essential oil and suddenly your memory of a traumatic event or stressor is gone and you have a new memory in its place. Instead, what I've experienced and what the data shows is that the memory itself will still be there, but the pain, shame, or trauma attached to the memory of the event is gone. You can remember without pain or fear or negativity.

Just using essential oils alone will have beneficial effects on our bodies, as does the simple process of engaging in conscious redirection of thought patterns to promote neurogenesis. However, the best and most effective way to facilitate the practice of "inner healing" is to engage the spirit, soul, and body in directed neuroplasticity with the addition of essential oils. This provides a combination of the physical, chemical, and quantum possibilities of essential oils to speed the

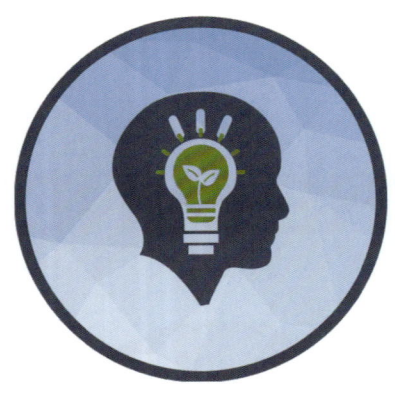

physical and quantum progression cleaning and redecorating your "house."

The decision to engage in the process of inner healing is yours and yours alone. It is with an act of your will that you consciously choose to engage in the clearing and restoration process. And it is precisely because it is an act of your will that there is power for healing. In proportion to your expectancy it will be done to you. There are a variety of methodologies that can be effective for processing stress, trauma, and overcoming blocks. Most of them can easily be combined with essential oils to increase their efficacy.

Regardless of what inner healing method you use, essential oils can be combined either aromatically, topically, or internally—depending on the desired outcome.

One of my favorite methods for using essential oils when doing an emotional release is to apply a few drops of the preferred oil(s) to the trauma point in the middle of the forehead and a few drops to the back of the head on the occipital bone near the foramen magnum—the opening to your brainstem (sometimes marked by a little notch at the base of your head). The subject then directly inhales by cupping hands over the nose and mouth, breathing in both nostrils together and then each nostril one at a time. This combined application is the fastest way to get the essential oil into the frontal lobe, limbic lobe, and brainstem.

After applying the oil, the subjects then puts one hand on the forehead and one over the heart. Then you repeat a simple phrase three times choosing to release the trauma behind the trapped emotion you're experiencing (even if it doesn't feel trapped or traumatic) and embracing the opposite experience.

In one sense, this is the most basic form of "cognitive behavioral therapy" as you unidentify with the old thought pattern and come into agreement with the new thought, by an act of your will. By your conscious choice to engage in the process of unidentifying with the toxic thought and agreeing with the new, healthy thought, what has occurred is your engaging in the neural dewiring and wiring process. Sometimes it will take days, weeks, months, or years to "clean and redecorate the house" and sometimes it can happen in a moment.

As your spirit and soul become realigned, your body follows suit and it manifests in your DNA. If you behold light, you will be filled with light. Just like we can't always isolate the sources of our stress, the emotions, trauma, and diseased states we experience don't happen in isolation either. The plants our essential oils are coming from live in an ecosystem, an environment with many factors like varying sunshine, amount of rainfall, soil conditions, environmental chemicals, and humans and animals. All of those conditions affect the plant in various ways and it responds to the biodynamic environment it's around.

Even so, your spirit, soul, and body are biodynamic. Not only is it important to not just treat symptoms, but to examine underlying structures, lifestyle choices, and the environment you are surrounded by. Your physical body, your mind, will, and emotions, and your spirit are all interconnected. It's possible that as you clear trauma, stress, or diseased states, other things will pop up that need to be dealt with. That's alright and very normal. You'll discover new doorways and there is grace for the process of illumination, cleaning, and restoring. It's important to listen to your spirit, soul, and body and respond to your needs and recognize this is a journey over time.

SEEDS

Over the years, I've discovered that often when we fight hopelessness, it's because we're believing a lie that nothing is going to change. As a result, we either white knuckle our way through with frustration and sheer grit or we resign ourselves to living life the way that it is now because we're too exhausted to do anything else. Neither of those options have to be in the cards for you.

I'm here to tell you that freedom is available. You are one who is destined to thrive. What you've known in the past doesn't have to be what the future holds. Sometimes healing is instantaneous and sometimes it's a process over time, but healing does come. I've experienced it and I've seen it in countless others and I know that it can be reality for you. In fact, it *is* reality for you. The healing may not have manifested yet in your life, but you are going to thrive and it can start today.

Healing is available for you, but it's not just for you. The beautiful thing about plants is that when they're next to each other in a field, one single plant effects everything around it. The nutrients emitted by one plant affect the entire ecosystem. My healing isn't just for me; my healing is available for you. Likewise, your healing as you obtain it isn't just for you. It's meant to be shared with the world as a beacon of hope to others that life can be new and is possible, in greater measure than ever before, in fresh ways, with vibrancy.

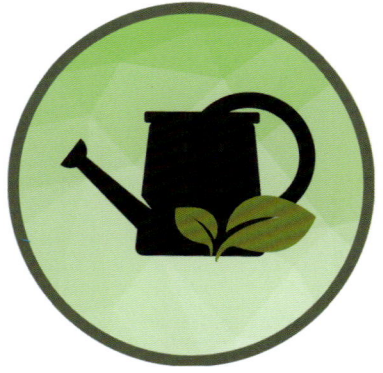

As you embark on each new day, fresh with possibilities and brimming with hope, may you know that you are worthy of receiving and all that you have need of will be provided. That is the nature of grace: it's the enabling power that causes you to thrive; it's living in the light and loving the freedom within. We are living beings who can't earn it; it's freely given. We open ourselves to receive it and sometimes, when we're desperate and broken and unaware of our need, grace meets us somewhere unexpectedly and profoundly. Because every breath is grace.

ESSENTIAL OILS TO AID YOUR BRAIN

BASIL *(Ocimum basilicum)*
Known to aid with anxiety, agitation, stress, challenging behaviors, and aids in recovery from mental exhaustion and burnout. Contains antispasmodic, anti-inflammatory, and muscle relaxant properties, in addition to antiviral and antibacterial functions. It may also help to restore olfaction where a loss of smell has occurred. *Note: avoid use if epileptic.

BERGAMOT *(Citrus aurantium bergamia)*
Calming agent that supports hormones, alleviates depression and can affect anxiety, agitation, stress, and challenging behaviors. *Note: Avoid applying to skin that will be exposed to sunlight or UV light within 36 hours.

CEDARWOOD *(Cedrus atlantica)*
Has been known to stimulate the limbic lobe, including the pineal gland and has been used traditionally in Ayurveda medicine for the treatment of central nervous system disorders. Antiepileptic and anxiolytic activity. Found to increase serotonin and noradrenaline levels of brain.

CLARY SAGE *(Salvia sclarea)*
It has been known to enhance the immune system, address skin issues, calm digestion and muscle spasms, balance hormones, and alleviate pain and inflammation. It is steam distilled from flowering plants and has a calming scent good for relieving stress. In recent studies, clary sage oil was found to be very effective in controlling cortisol levels in women.

CLOVE *(Syzgium aromaticum)*
Clove contains a high amount of eugenol, known for its analgesic effects. Has been known for centuries for its antimicrobial, antifungal, antiviral, analgesic, and anti-inflammatory properties (among others). It can act as a mental stimulant and also can encourage sleep and feelings of rest. It has also been studied for its effect on the thyroid and its effect on memory, cognition and altering mood. *Note: Caution should be used if combined with Warfarin, aspirin, etc. as anticoagulant properties can be enhanced.

COPAIBA *(Copaifera officinalis, C. reticulata)*
Known for its anti-inflammatory, antiseptic, and neuroprotective properties. Researchers found that copaiba was neuroprotective by modulating inflammatory response following an acute damage to the central nervous system. It contains high amounts of β-Caryophyllene, the first known "dietary cannabinoid", which has now been shown to be directly beneficial for cerebral ischemia, anxiety and depression and Alzheimer-like disease types

EUCALYPTUS *(Eucalyptus citriodora, E. bicostata, E. dives, E. globulus, E. polybractea, E. radiata, E. staigeriana)*
There are multiple varieties of eucalyptus essential oil available and though there are powerful crossover properties as an antiviral, anti-inflammatory, antifungal, and mucolytic research has shown that Eucalyptus citriodora leaf extract may have a beneficial effect in affecting Parkinson's disease and other degenerative neurological conditions. Eucalyptus oils have been used to regulate and activate the various systems like nervous system for neuralgia, headache and physical weakness and has been known as an antidepressant as it promotes clarity of mind.

FRANKINCENSE *(Boswellia sacra, B. carterii, B. frereana, B. serrata)*
Frequently used for uplifting emotions, aiding cognitive function, facilitating muscle relaxation, significantly reversing the age-induced deterioration of memory, improving cognitive performance, and promoting cellular health. Boswellia resin contains incensole acetate, a constituent that has been found to modulate the hypothalamic–pituitary–adrenal (HPA) axis and influence hippocampal gene expression. Researchers believe this can lead to beneficial behavioral effects and supports its potential as a novel treatment of depressive-like disorders. Another study found that Boswellia resin acts as a major anti-inflammatory agent to help the brain following major head trauma and protects against ischemic (stroke) neuronal damage. This study suggests that the anti-inflammatory and neuroprotective activities of incensole acetate may serve as a novel therapeutic treatment for restoring blood flow after a stroke or injury.

GERANIUM *(Pelargonium graveolens)*
Useful for the release of negative memories and nervous tension. It helps to balance emotions and the aroma is uplifting to the nervous system and has been known to help balance hormones and improve circulation. Researchers have found that inhaling geranium essential oil led to subjects reporting significantly lower levels of anxiety. Uses for geranium essential oil have reportedly included the treatment of inflammatory and pain associated ailments (i.e., headache, neuralgia), nervous system-related ailments (i.e., restlessness, nervousness, anxiety anger, frustration, emotional upsets).

LAVENDER *(Lavandula angustifolia)*
Lavender, sometimes known as the "Swiss army knife" of essential oils because of the variety of uses, has been shown to affect all five of the main cognitive functions: alertness, attention, cognition, memory, and emotional regulation. It has been shown to have main properties acting as an analgesic, antidepressant, anticonvulsant, anxiolytic, calming, hypnotic, relaxing, sedative. Researchers have found that lavender essential oil not only helps people feel more relaxed, but they also had more mental focus when performing math computations after inhalation. Researchers found that lavender odorants were associated with reduced mental stress and increased arousal rate. Can be wonderful to help with generalized emotional distress as well as acute symptoms of stress and can help in overcoming anxiety and depression.

LEMON *(Citrus limon)*
Effective for boosting the immune system, but recent research has also arisen in how it can improve productivity, positively decrease anxiety, boost self-esteem, and can positively affect learning. One study in particular found that lemon oil can have an anxiolytic, antidepressant-like effect that reduces distress by modulating the systems in the brain that produce GABA, serotonin, and dopamine. Another study found evidence to strongly support the hypothesis that oxidative stress in the hippocampus can occur during neurodegenerative diseases, but that lemon could have a strong protective effect as an antioxidant. *Note: Avoid applying to skin that will be exposed to sunlight or UV light within 24 hours. **Note: Orange (Citrus sinensis), Lime (Citrus latifolia or C. aurantifolia Swingle) and other citrus essential oils may have similar effects on the CNS as lemon due in part to their high limonene content, but are less researched.

MELISSA *(Melissa officinalis)*
Melissa has been known to help with promoting feelings of calm and aiding with sleep and throughout history was used to treat migraines, neuroses and hysteria. It has been reported to be a CNS depressant, analgesic, sedative, cholinergic, and antioxidative. It has also been researched highly (in addition to lavender) for its use in patients with dementia.

OREGANO *(Origanum vulgare)*
Powerful for its anti-aging, anti-inflammatory, antioxidant, anti-bacterial, antinoiceptive, radio-protective, and immune stimulating properties. One study found that oregano may possess antinociceptive (the blocking of detection of a painful or injurious stimulus by sensory neurons) activity in a dose-dependent manner that might be mediated, at least in part, by both GABA receptors. Oregano has also been shown to be beneficial in aiding the gut and acting as an anti-parasitic, which may have positive connotations on the gut-brain connection. *Note: Caution — oregano is high in phenols and therefore may cause irritation to the nasal membranes or skin if inhaled directly from the diffuser or applied neat.

PEPPERMINT *(Mentha piperita)*
Known to contain anti-inflammatory, antibacterial, anti-viral, anti-fungal, and antiparasitic properties as well as acting as a digestive stimulant and pain reliever. Researchers have found that inhaling peppermint can increase attention, focus, and performance during mental tasks. Studies have shown peppermint to have awakening effects resulting in decreased alpha and beta activities and increased alertness. Other studies have shown peppermint to effect emotions by reducing fatigue and improving mood. *Note: Avoid contact with eyes, mucus membranes, sensitive skin, or fresh wounds or burns. Use caution (some argue it's not recommended) on infants younger than 18 months of age.

ROMAN CHAMOMILE *(Anthemis nobilis)*
Known for its relaxant, anti-spasmodic, anti-inflammatory, antiparasitic, anti-bacterial, and anesthetic properties. One study found that an aromatherapy massage including chamomile

exerted positive effects on anxiety and self-esteem. It is thought that because of its calming properties, roman chamomile may be beneficial in alleviating depression, insomnia, nervous tension, and stress as well balancing emotions.

ROSE *(Rosa damascena)*
Known to have anti-inflammatory, antioxidant, anxiolytic, heptoprotective properties as well as serving as a relaxant, immunomodulating and serving to protect DNA. Some research has shown rose to be hypnotic, anticonvulsant, anti-depressant, anti-anxiety, analgesic effects, and perform nerve growth. Several studies confirm that rose inhibits the reactivity of the hypothalamus and pituitary systems and can suppress the reactivity of central nervous system. *Note: *Rosa damascena* (high in citronellol) is different from the Moroccan variety, *Rosa centifolia* (high in phenyl ethanol) and have differences not only in color and aroma, but in therapeutic benefit.

ROSEMARY *(Rosmarinus officinalis CT Cineole)*
Known for its variety of properties including: antibacterial, antifungal, anti-bacterial antidepressant, and enhances mental clarity and concentration. Studies have shown that rosemary increased alertness, produced a significant enhancement of performance for overall quality of memory, and can have positive effects on anxiety and self-esteem. Other studies have shown rosemary to help balance emotions by reducing anxiety and feelings of depression. *Note: Do not use on children under 4 years of age. Do not use rosemary for high blood pressure if already taking ACE inhibitor prescription drugs.

SAGE *(Salvia officinalis)*
Known to contain antibacteria, antiviral, anti-inflammatory, antioxidant, antifungal, and anxi-olytic properties in addition to assisting in regulating hormones. Studies have shown sage to have a cholinergic, stimulatory, GABAergic, and antioxidant effects on the central nervous system. Other studies have shown that sage might be a useful remedy for patients with dementia. *Note: In (very) high does, thujone can be neurotoxic. Avoid if epileptic or on persons with high blood pressure. **Note: Spanish Sage (Salvia lavandulifolia) has also been researched for its neuroprotective properties against brain cell death and age-related memory loss.

SANDALWOOD *(Santalum album)*
Known to be extremely useful for removing negative information from cells and stimulating the limbic system. One study found sandalwood beneficial for enhancing memory. Other studies have found that sandalwood promotes feelings of relaxation resulting in subjects feeling more comfortable with alpha 1 decreased at parietal and posterior temporal regions as well as improvements in productivity due to its sedative effect. Researchers have also found that not only can sandalwood be calming to the nervous system, but the results can linger even up to 24 hours after the stressor was presented.

VALERIAN *(Valeriana officinalis)*
Research has shown that the sesquiterpenes in valerian act in a sedative, tranquilizing, and antispasmodic way to the central nervous system as has been used in treatments of insomnia and anxiety. Studies are now showing that the active valerenic acid within interacts with the GABAergic system, a mechanism of action similar to the benzodiazepine drugs. It serves the body by calming, grounding, promoting feelings of relaxation, and emotional balancing.

VETIVER *(Vetiveria zizanioides)*
Known for its antiseptic, antispasmodic and historically anti-inflammatory properties as well as a relaxant and circulatory stimulant and contains calming, nerve tonic, sedative, and uplifting properties. Researchers have also found that vetiver can enhance memory and learning activity.

YLANG YLANG *(Cananga odorata)*
Has been known to be involved in mood regulation and regulates heartbeat in addition to its antispasmodic, vasodilating, anti-inflammatory, antiparasitic capabilities. Ylang ylang has been shown to increase positive energy and focus of thoughts, restore confidence, peace, and decrease alertness as it promoted feelings of tranquility. *Note: Use sparingly if you have low blood pressure.

 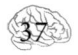

ESSENTIAL OILS FOR BRAIN CONDITIONS

This "cheat sheet" is not meant to diagnose, treat, or prevent any disease state or condition. Rather, it's meant as a quick glance tool to help accompany your practical usage. The essential oils below are listed in order of their effectiveness for the particular outcome desired.

There are three keys which need to be remembered before you reach for an oil:

1. Keep in mind that to support the brain, you'll want to support it's structure <u>and</u> function. To best support the structure, a consistent intake of clean water, healthy diet, exercise, antioxidants (such as the wolfberry!), healthy fats, vitamins, and minerals should be consumed regularly. Adding oils <u>and</u> supporting the structure will help you see better results in brain function.

2. Remember each body and situation are different. This list is not comprehensive, nor are these the only oils you should be using. Depending on each situation and the ecosystem of the individual, you might need to change oils or protocols. Many essential oils will contain some crossover properties. So if you don't have "the right oil", grab another one in the same family, or whatever you have nearby, and as you combine your intention with the oil, it becomes a "packet of possibilities".

3. The oils listed here are single essential oils only. Blends of various single essential oils can be even more effective because of the synergistic effect of the chemical components at work at one time. You also can layer single essential oils during application for a similar effect to using an essential oil blend.

ADD / ADHD
- VETIVER
- LAVENDER
- CEDARWOOD
- SANDALWOOD
- CARDAMOM
- PEPPERMINT

ALS
- ROSEMARY
- SANDALWOOD
- FRANKINCENSE
- HELICHRYSUM
- CYPRESS
- SAGE

ALZHEIMER'S
- FRANKINCENSE
- MELISSA
- CEDARWOOD
- SANDALWOOD
- HELICHRYSUM
- VETIVER

ANXIETY
- LAVENDER
- YLANG YLANG
- BLUE SPRUCE
- ROMAN CHAMOMILE
- PALO SANTO
- FRANKINCENSE

AUTISM
- VETIVER
- PATCHOULI
- LAVENDER
- SANDALWOOD
- EUCALYPTUS GLOBULUS
- MELISSA
- CEDARWOOD

BIPOLAR
- ROSE
- PALO SANTO
- FRANKINCENSE
- VETIVER

COMA

- VALERIAN
- VETIVER
- SANDALWOOD
- BLUE CYPRESS
- BLACK PEPPER

CONCENTRATION

- PEPPERMINT
- BASIL
- JADE LEMON
- LEMON
- LIME
- ROSEMARY

CONFUSION

- CEDARWOOD
- BLACK SPRUCE
- PEPPERMINT
- SACRED FRANKINCENSE

DEPRESSION

- SACRED FRANKINCENSE
- FRANKINCENSE
- BLUE SPRUCE
- COPAIBA
- PALO SANTO
- LEMON

FEAR

- BLUE SPRUCE
- PALO SANTO
- CYPRESS
- ROMAN CHAMOMILE
- GERANIUM

LEARNING DISABILITY

- SACRED FRANKINCENSE
- FRANKINCENSE
- VETIVER
- CEDARWOOD
- LAVENDER

MEMORY

- ROSEMARY
- PEPPERMINT
- CARDAMOM
- BASIL
- VETIVER
- PALO SANTO

MENTAL FATIGUE

- SACRED FRANKINCENSE
- FRANKINCENSE
- ROSEMARY
- VETIVER
- CEDARWOOD

OCD (OBSESSIVENESS)

- CLARY SAGE
- OCOTEA
- PALO SANTO
- CYPRESS
- GERANIUM
- HELICHRYSUM

PANIC

- BLUE SPRUCE
- BERGAMOT
- BALSAM FIR
- ROMAN CHAMOMILE
- MYRRH
- FRANKINCENSE

PARALYSIS

- PEPPERMINT
- LEMONGRASS
- GERANIUM
- CYPRESS
- GINGER
- PALO SANTO

PARKINSON'S

- HELICHRYSUM
- LAVENDER
- PEPPERMINT
- CEDARWOOD
- MYRRH
- SACRED FRANKINCENSE

POST TRAUMATIC STRESS DISORDER (PTSD)

- FRANKINCENSE
- LAVENDER
- CEDARWOOD
- PALO SANTO
- VALERIAN

SCHIZOPHRENIA

- CARDAMOM
- CEDARWOOD
- VETIVER
- MELISSA
- ROSEMARY
- BLUE SPRUCE

SEIZURES

- SACRED FRANKINCENSE
- FRANKINCENSE
- PALO SANTO
- EUCALYPTUS BLUE
- COPAIBA

*Caution: Avoid Sage essential oil

STRESS

- BLUE SPRUCE
- ROMAN CHAMOMILE
- YLANG YLANG
- ANGELICA
- FRANKINCENSE
- LAVENDER

STROKE

HEMORRHAGIC	THROMBOTIC
• CYPRESS	• HELICHRYSUM
• CISTUS	• FRANKINCENSE
• HELICHRYSUM	• CISTUS
• NUTMEG	• NUTMEG
• SANDALWOOD	• CYPRESS
• FRANKINCENSE	• SANDALWOOD

TOURETTES

- PALO SANTO
- SANDALWOOD
- ROSE
- FRANKINCENSE
- HELICHRYSUM

TRAUMA

- SANDALWOOD
- FRANKINCENSE
- VALERIAN
- BLACK SPRUCE
- GERANIUM
- HELICHRYSUM
- LAVENDER

TRAUMATIC BRAIN INJURY (CONCUSSION)

- COPAIBA
- FRANKINCENSE
- CYPRESS
- VETIVER
- CEDARWOOD
- SANDALWOOD
- HELICHRYSUM
- LAVENDER
- PALO SANTO
- PEPPERMINT
- PATCHOULI